Flowers from magical garden

This coloring book for adults contains swirls style illustrations
representing floral compositions. The twenty-one designs are
of various difficulty levels.
The images are printed on the fronts of pages only, so you don't
need to worry about bleed-through if you choose to use markers.
BONUS: The book includes also the E-mail for receive a discount
for the following books! Happy Coloring! magicstarclub@gmail.com
Thanks!
Valentyn Tykhomirov

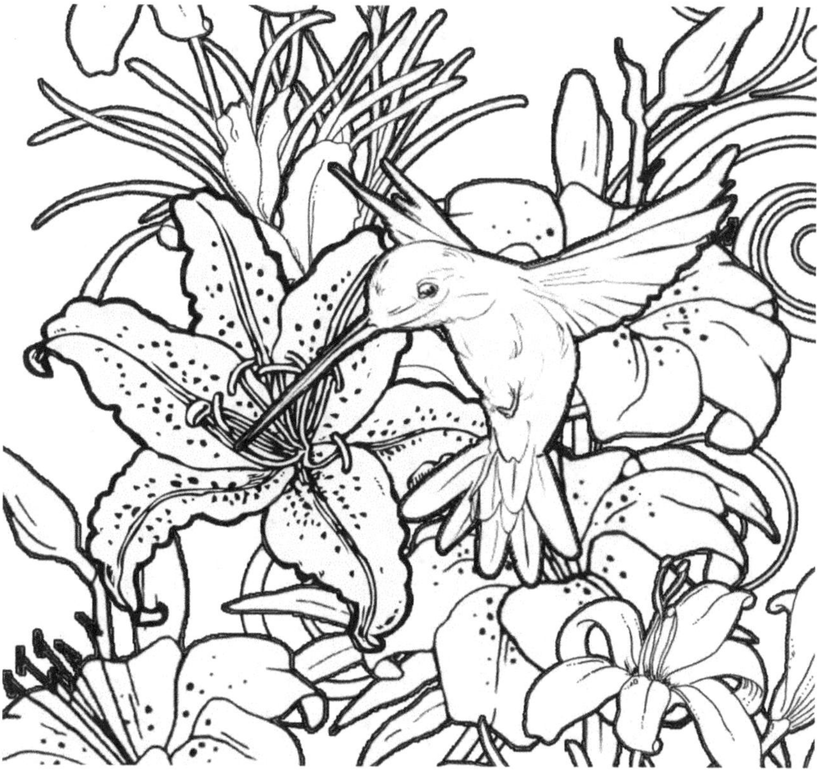

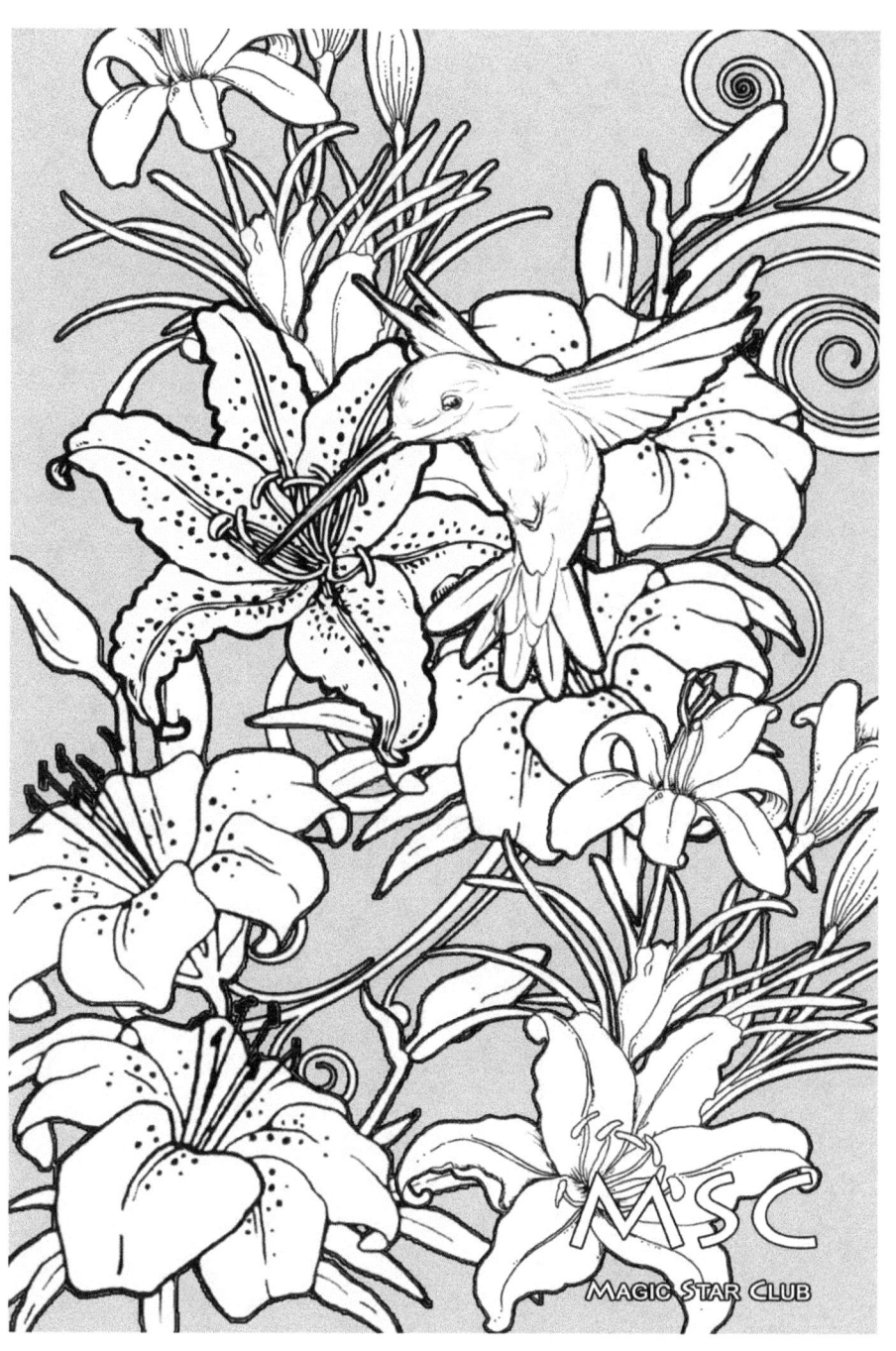

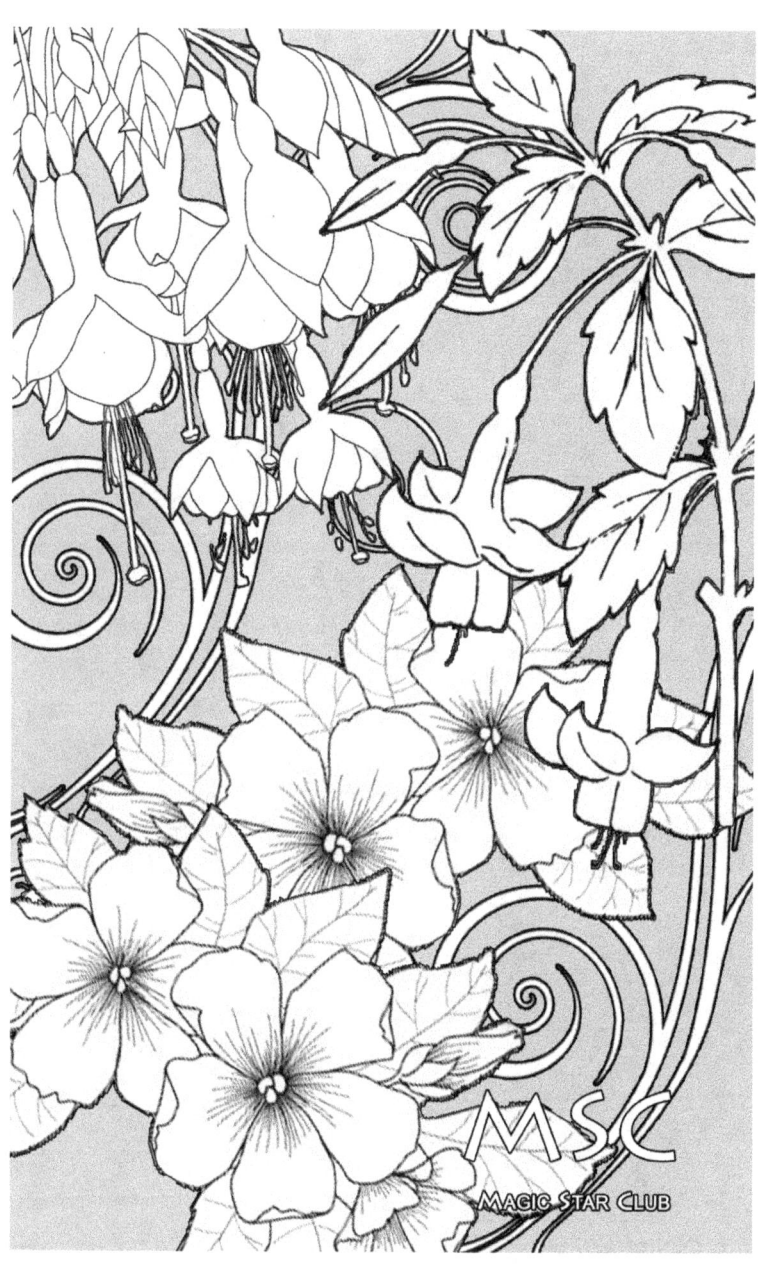

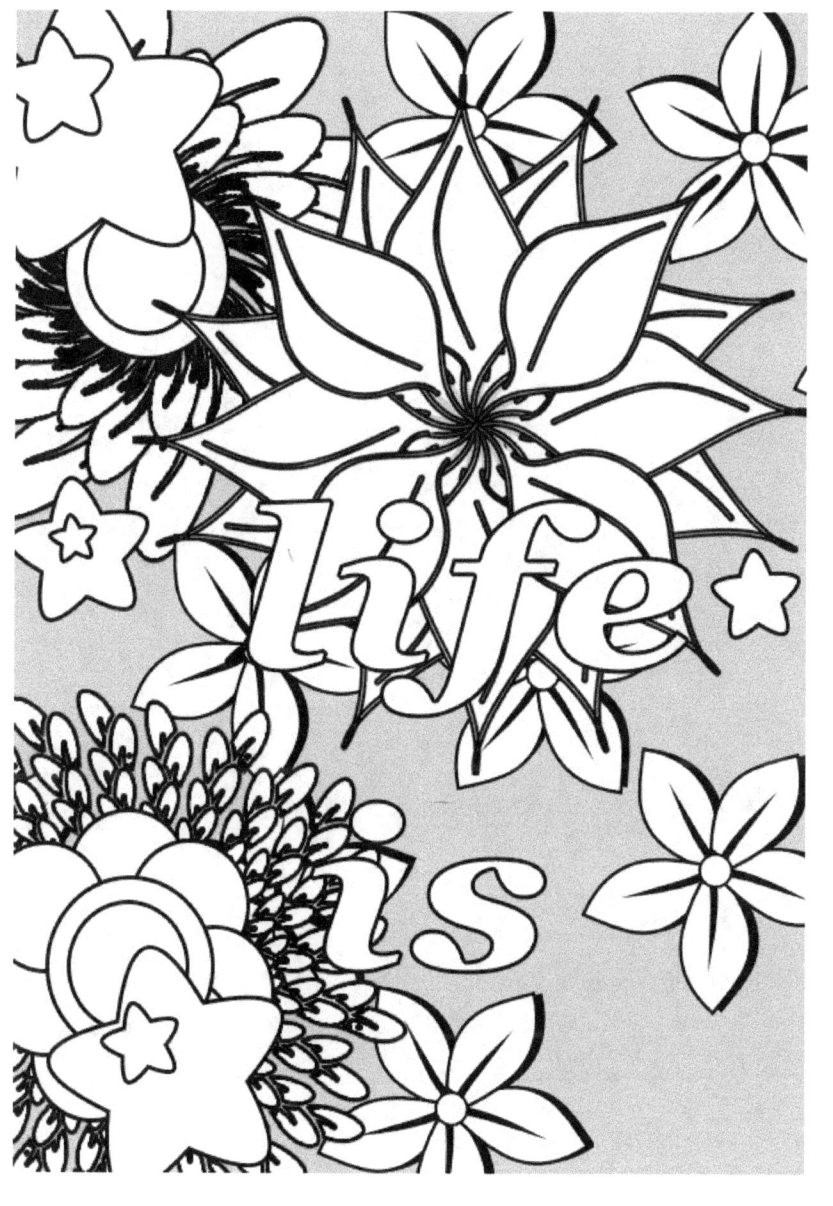

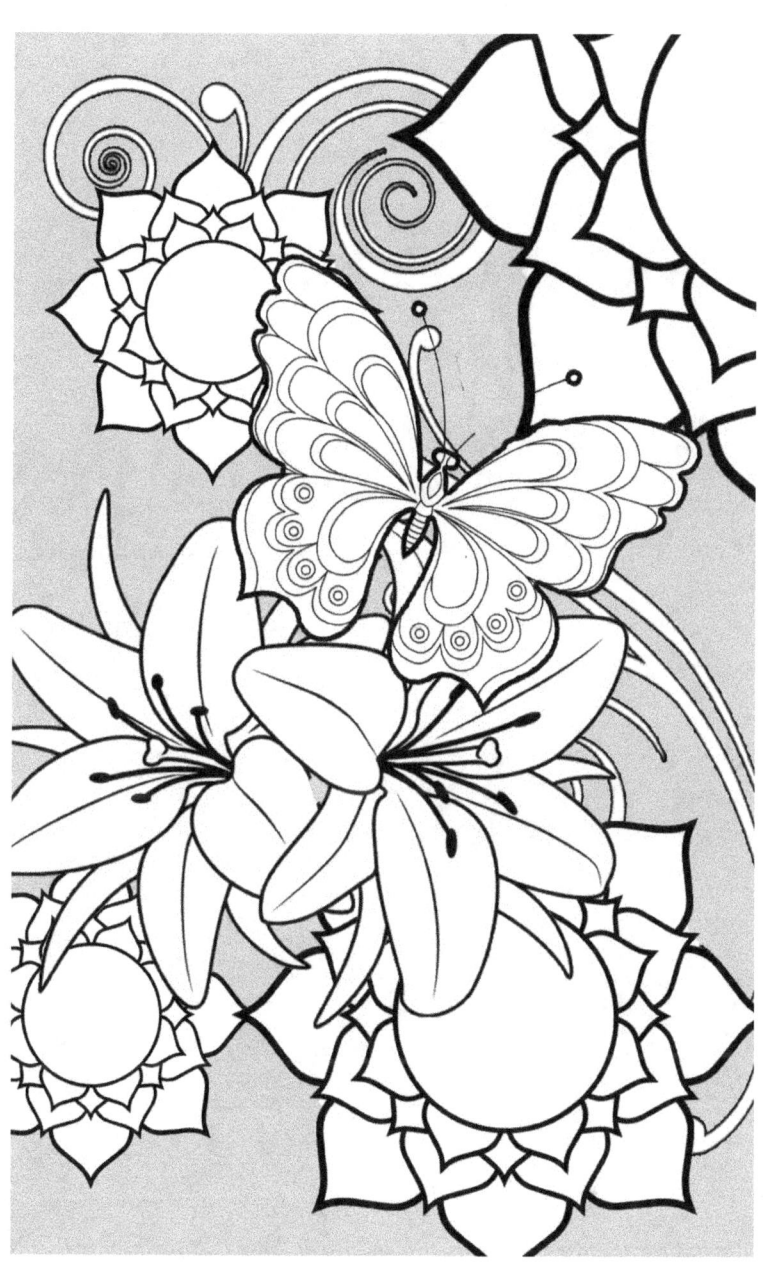

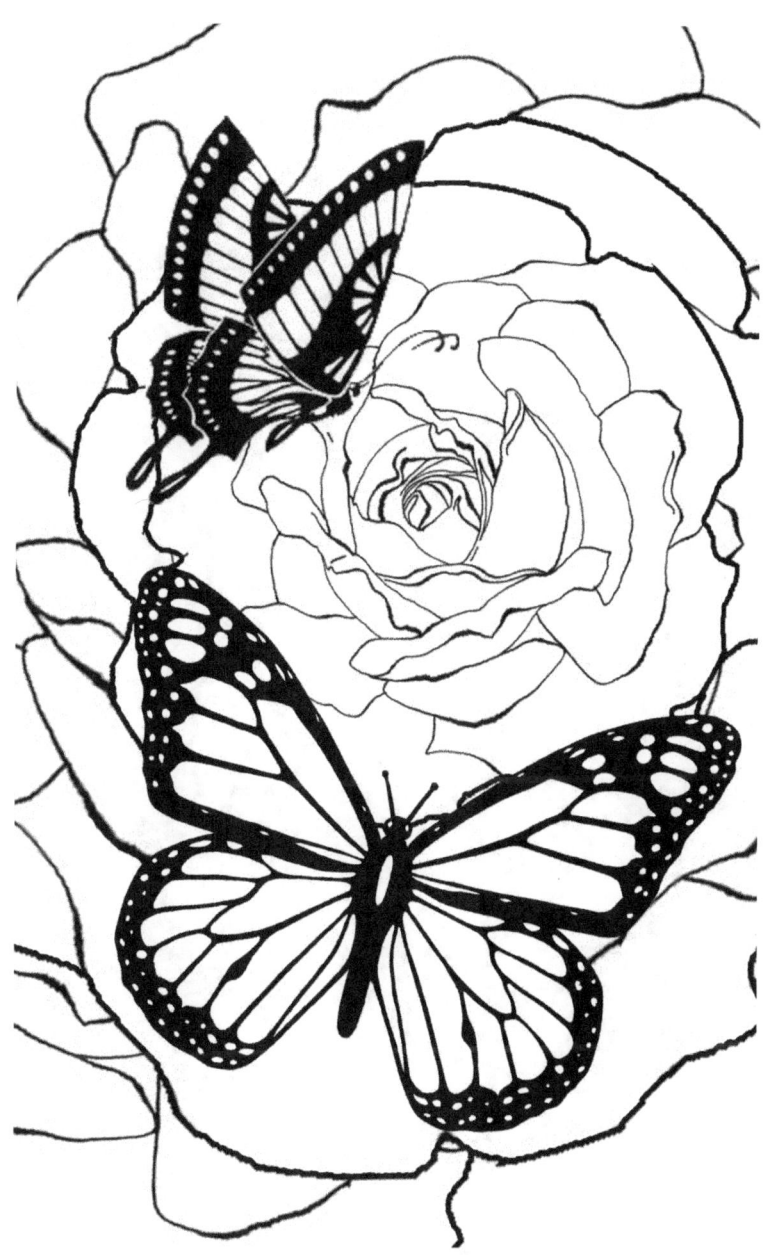

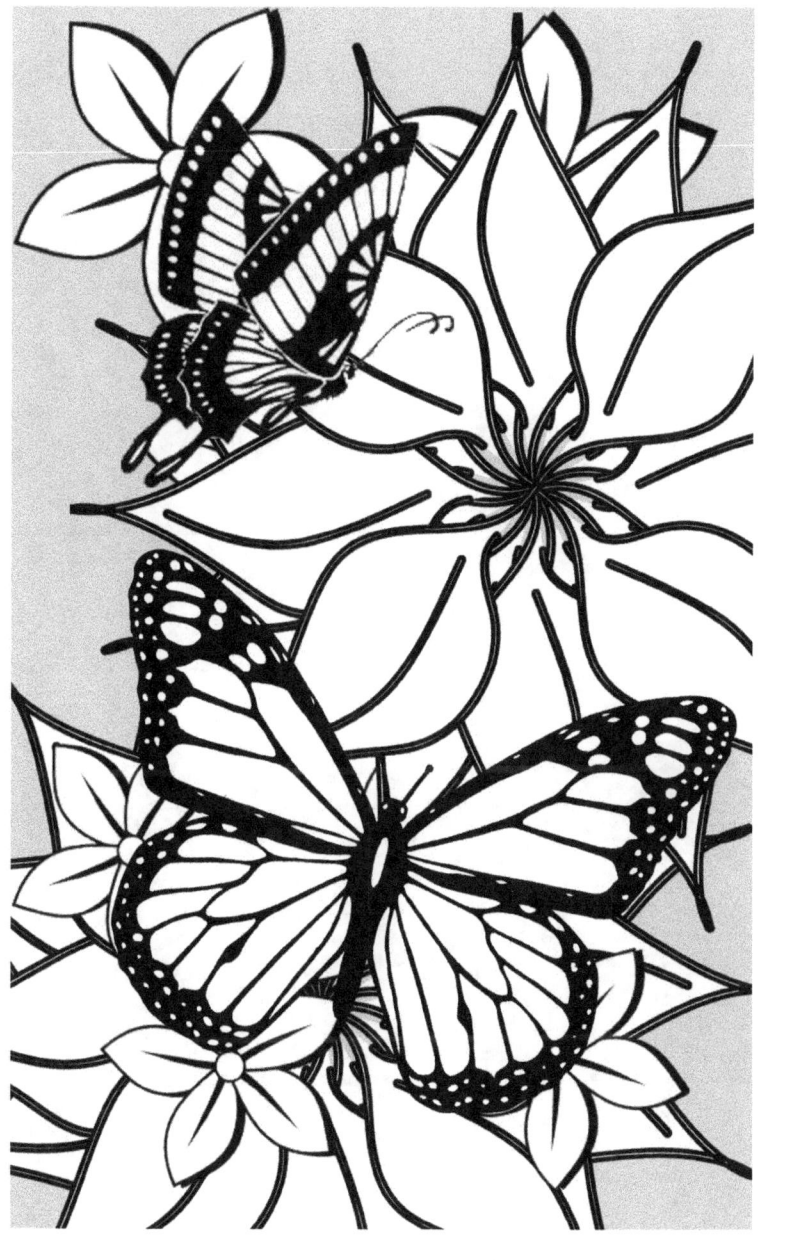

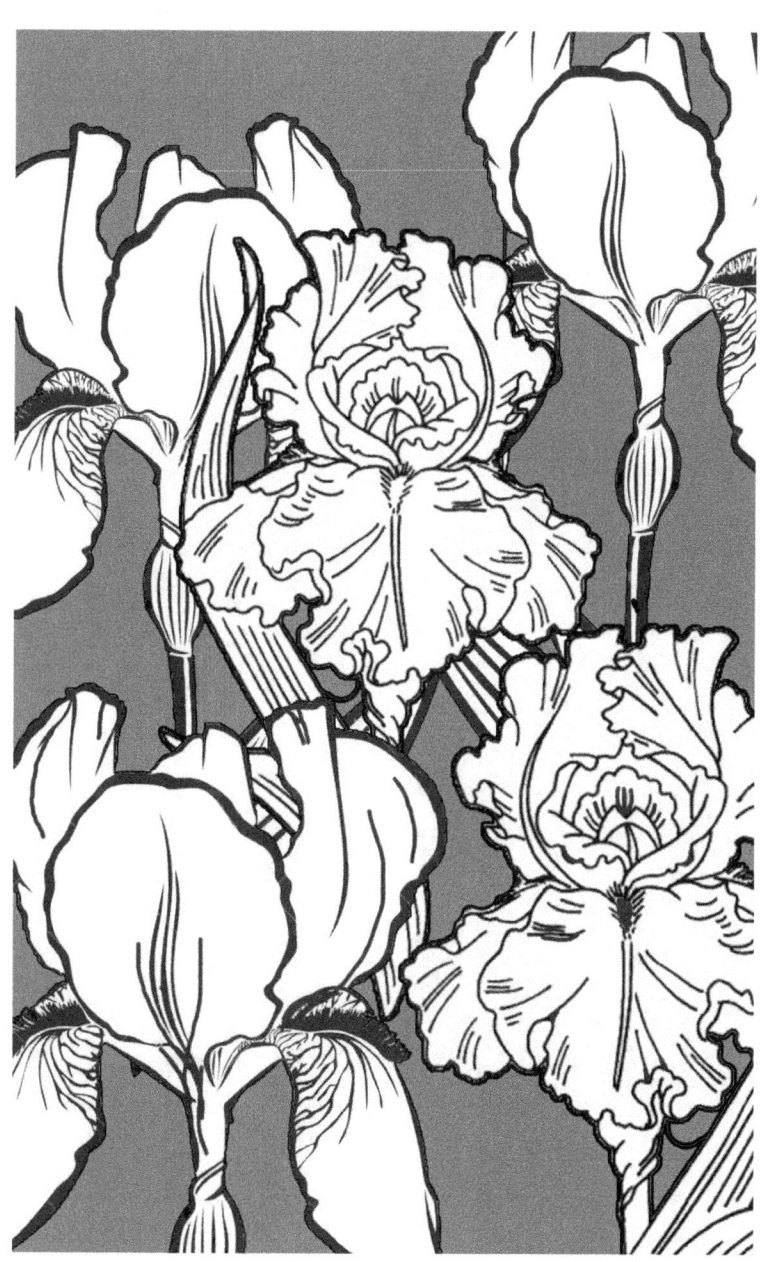

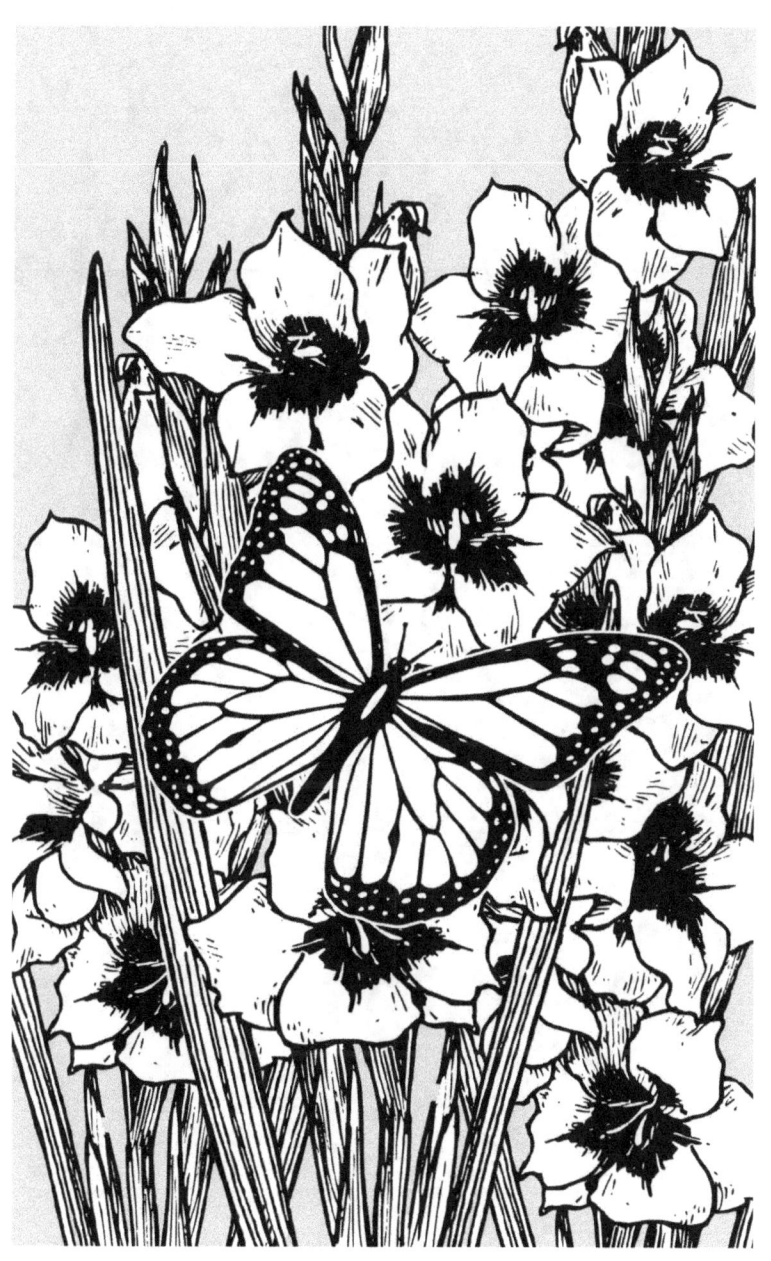

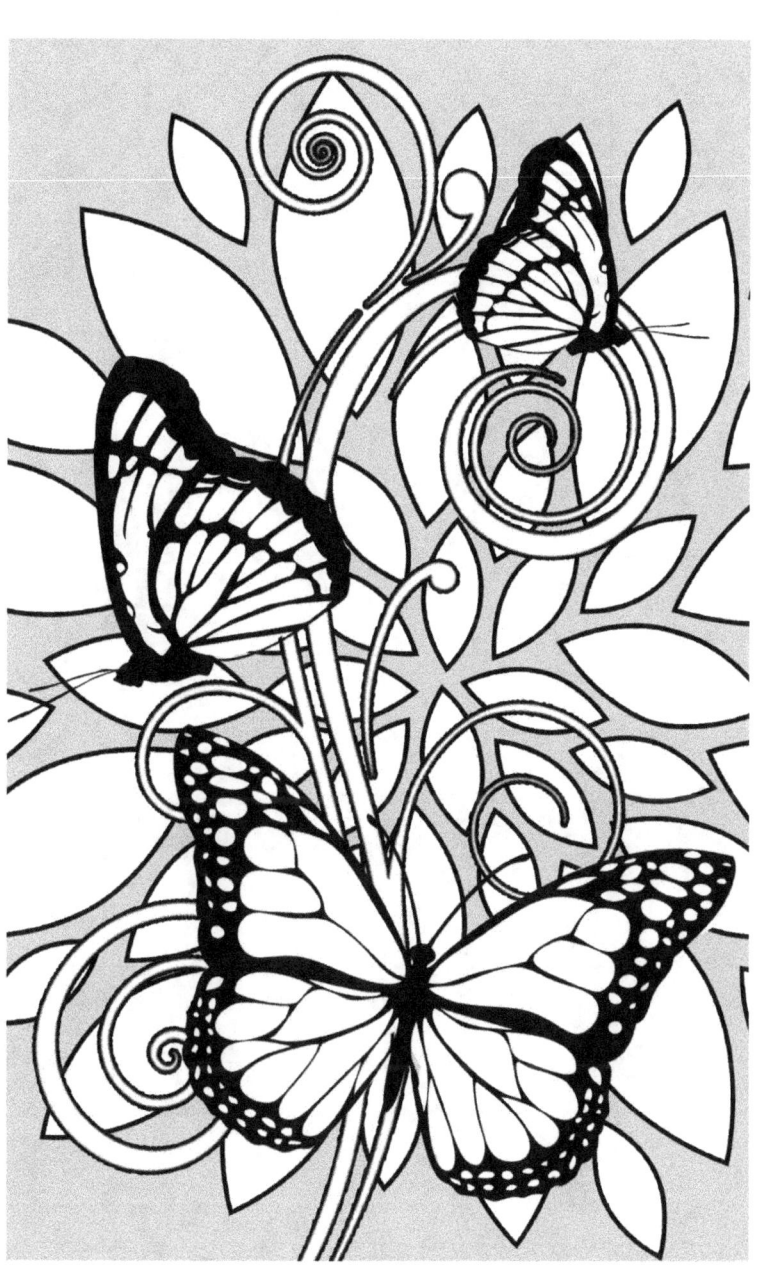

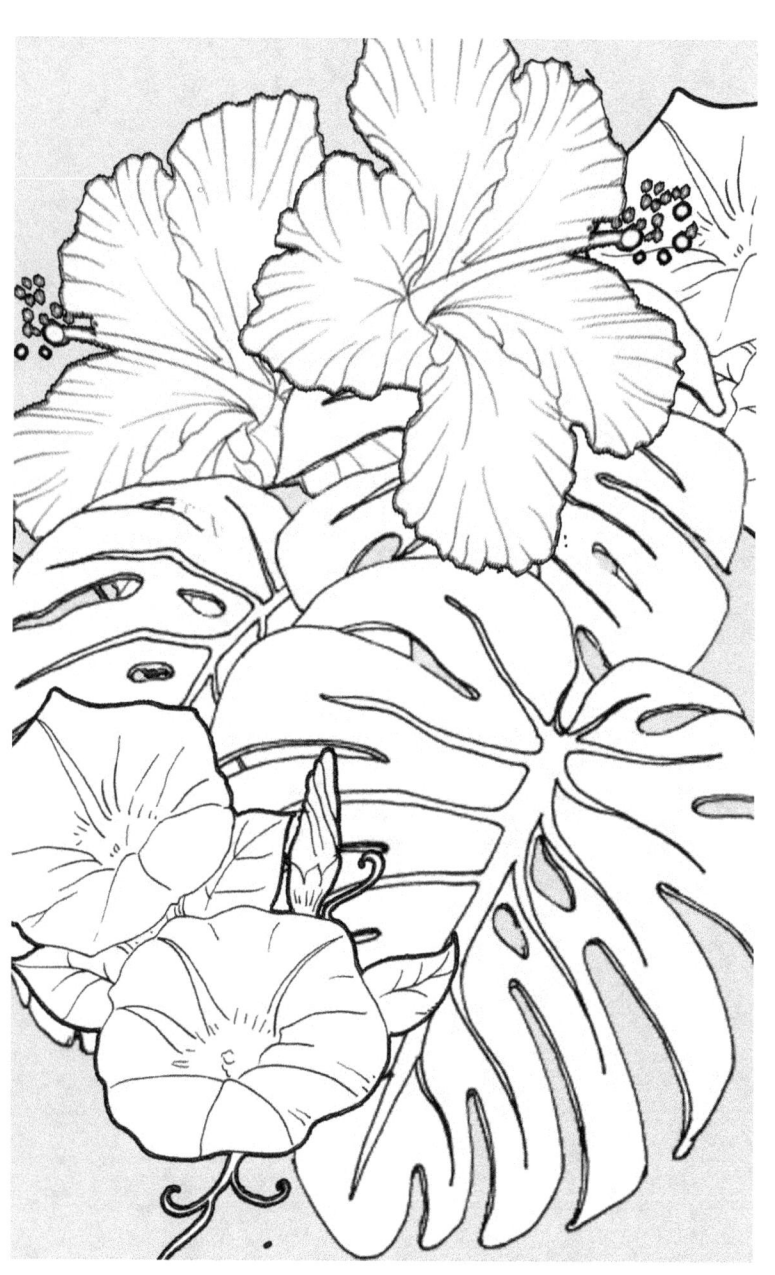

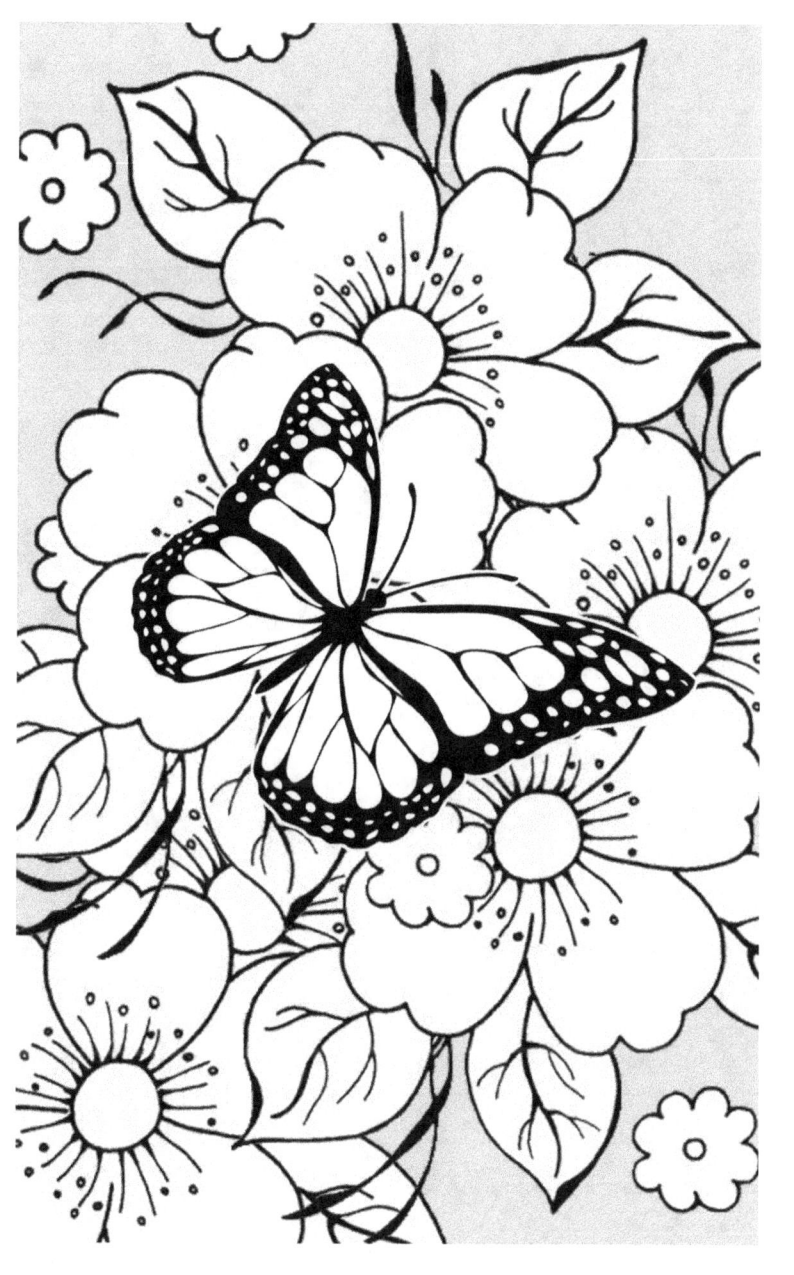

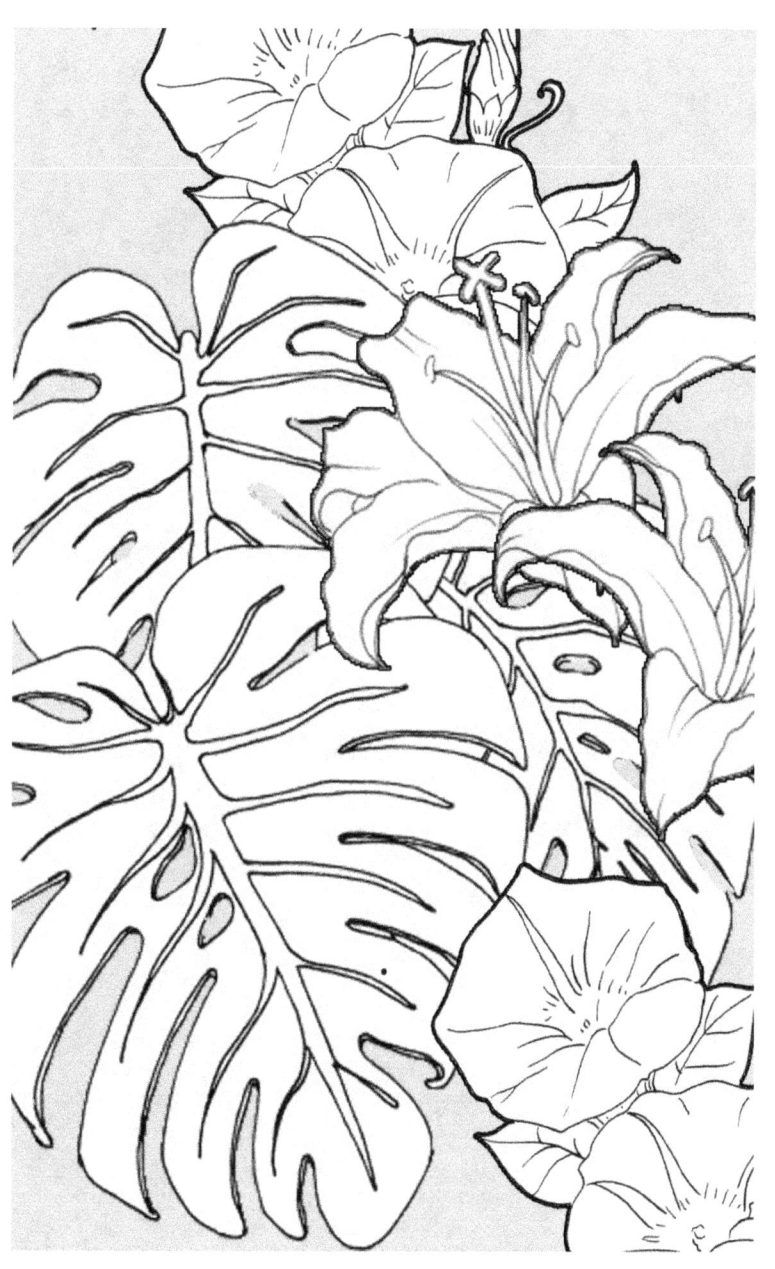

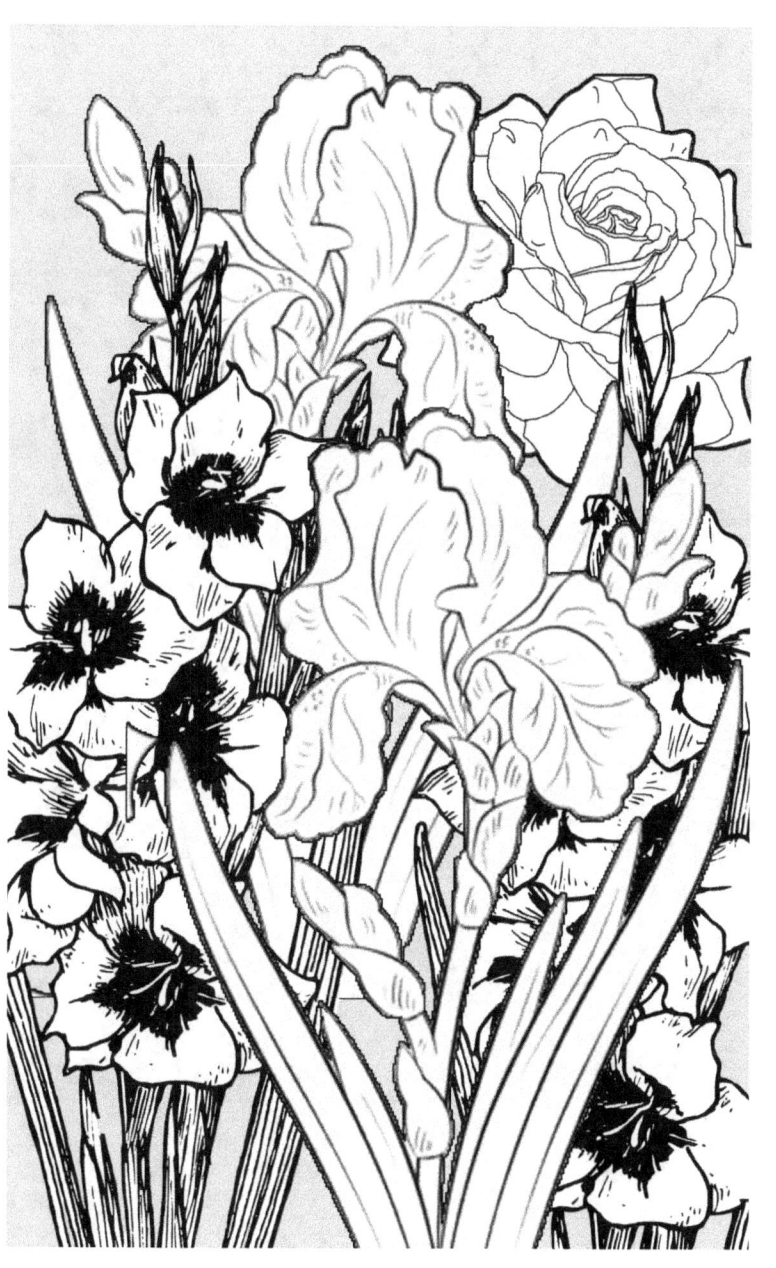

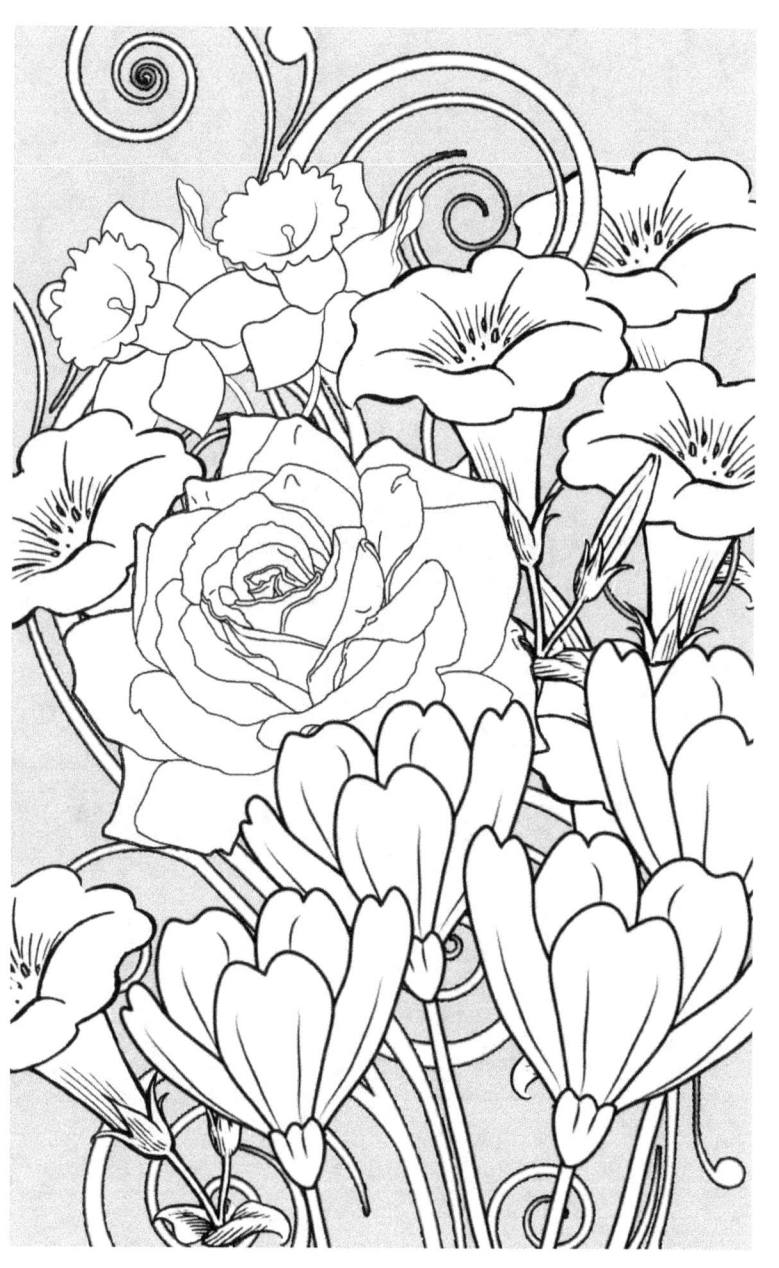

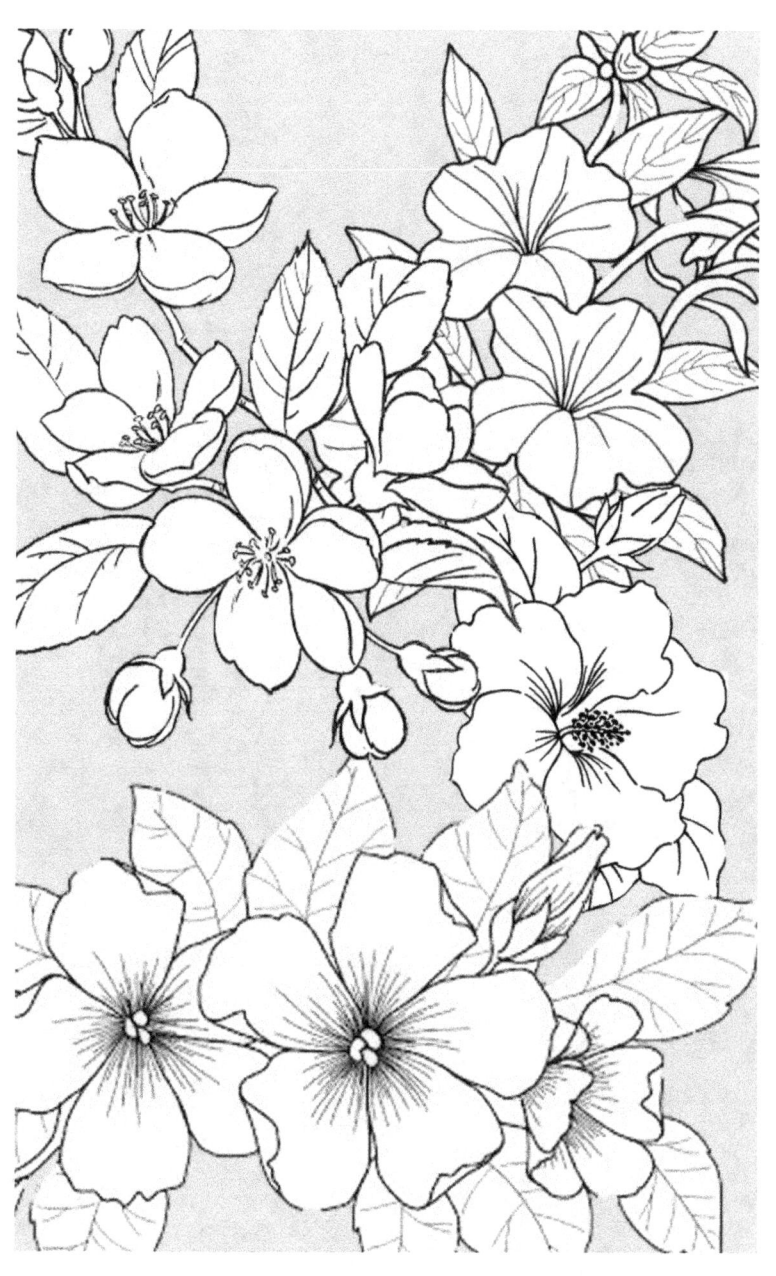

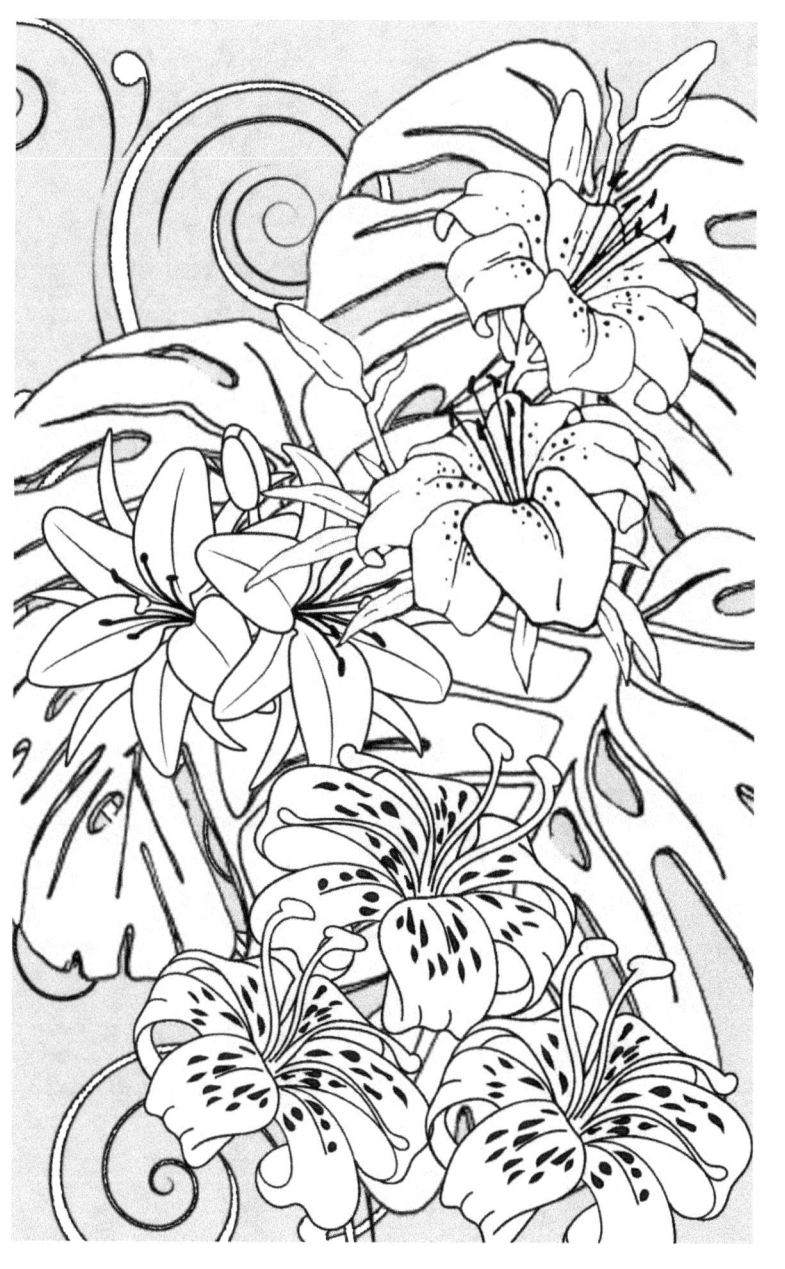

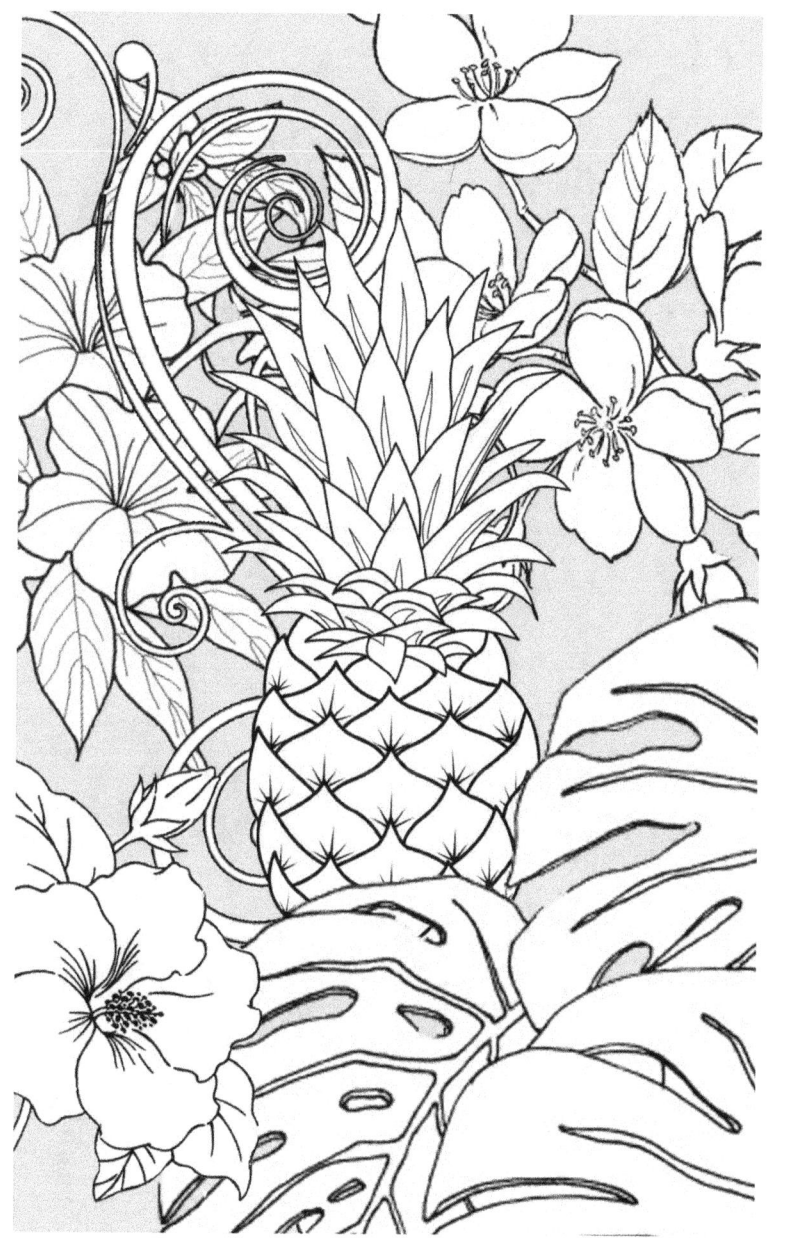

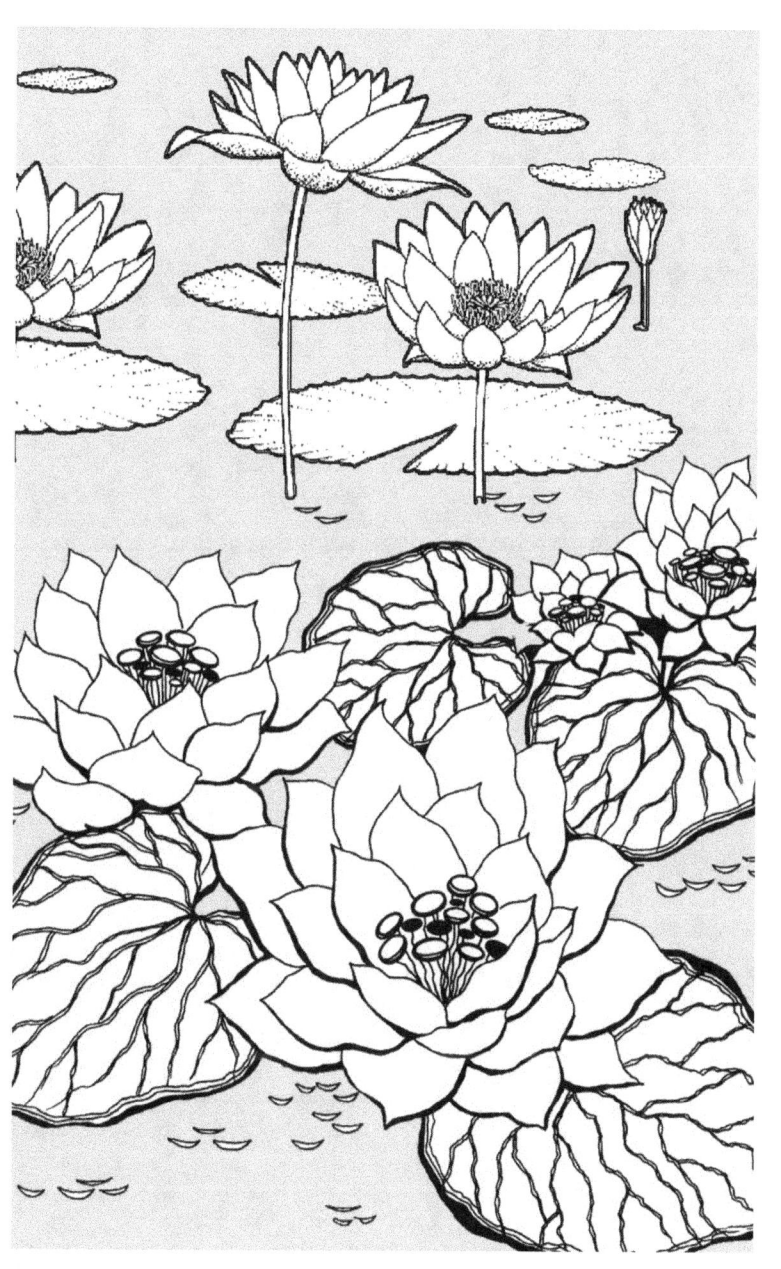

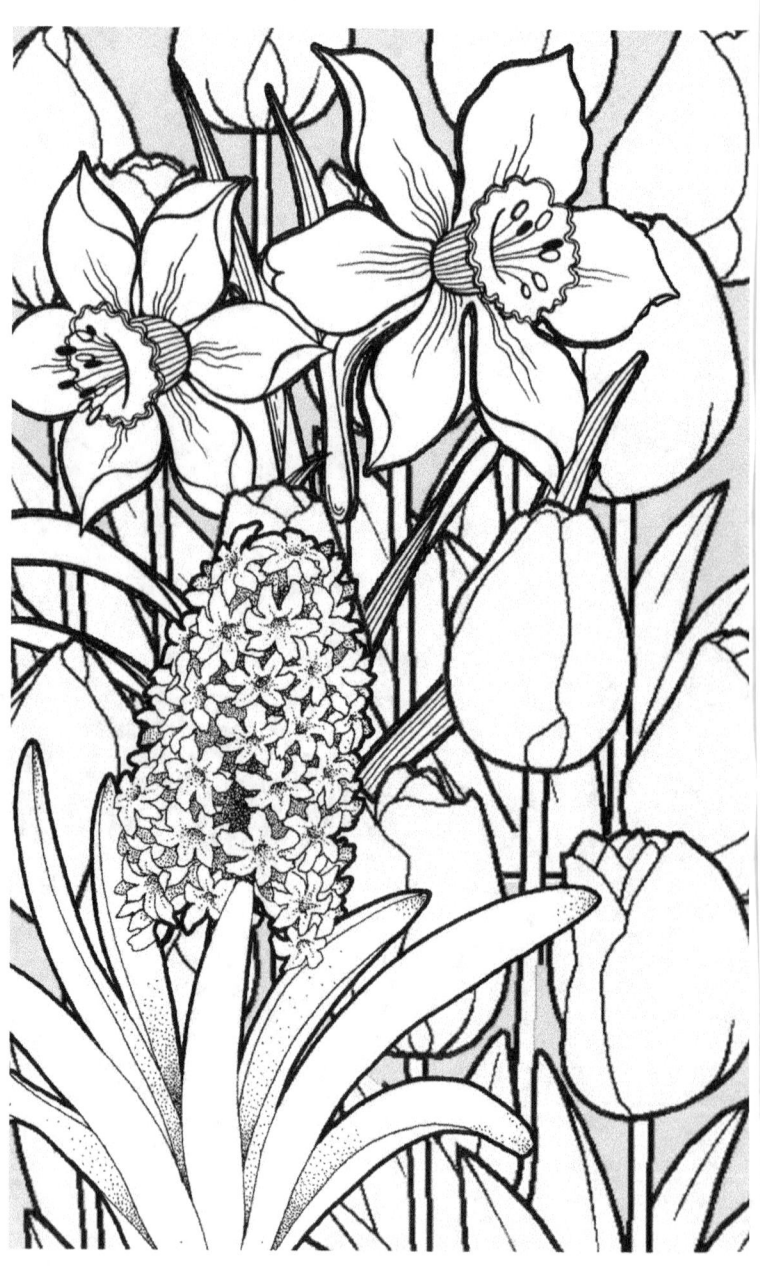

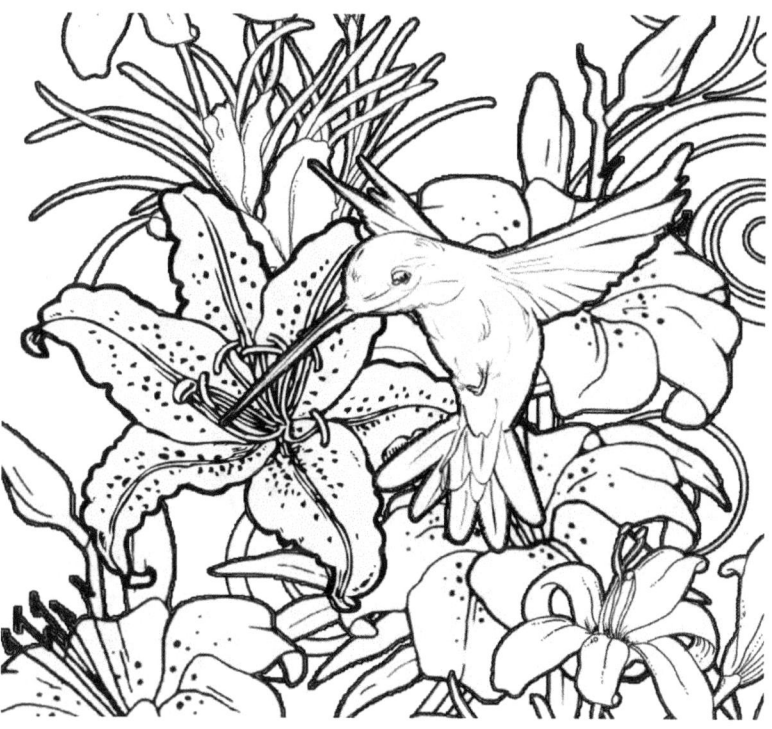

www.ingramcontent.com/pod-product-compliance
Lightning Source LLC
Chambersburg PA
CBHW072023280526
45788CB00007B/2648